Cobalt 3

OTHER BOOKS BY KEVIN ROBERTS

Cariboo Fishing Notes (Beau Geste Press 1972) poems

West Country (Oolichan 1975) poems

Stonefish (Oolichan 1978) poems

Deep Line (Harbour Publishing 1982) poems

Nanoose Bay Suite (Oolichan 1984) poems

Picking the Morning Colour (Oolichan 1985) short stories

Tears in a Glass Eye (Douglas & McIntyre 1989) novel

Red Centre Journal (Wakefield Press 1992) poems

Cobalt 3

Kevin Roberts
poems

RONSDALE PRESS

COBALT 3
Copyright © 2000 Kevin Roberts

RONSDALE PRESS
3350 West 21st Avenue
Vancouver, B.C., Canada
V6S 1G7

Set in New Baskerville: 11 pt on 13.5
Typesetting: Julie Cochrane
Printing: Hignell Printing, Winnipeg, Manitoba
Cover Design: Julie Cochrane
Back Cover Author Photo: Jim Sabiston

The cover photo is the biopsy of the author's cancer cell, courtesy of Dr. J. Whitelaw

Ronsdale Press wishes to thank the Canada Council for the Arts, the Government of Canada through the Book Publishing Industry Development Program (BPIDP), and the Province of British Columbia through the British Columbia Arts Council for their support of its publishing program.

CANADIAN CATALOGUING IN PUBLICATION DATA

Roberts, Kevin, 1940–
  Cobalt 3

  Poems.
  ISBN 0-921870-73-6

  I. Title. II. Title: Cobalt three.
PS8585.O297C62 2000   C811'.54   C99-911254-6
PR9199.3.R5312C62 2000

for
D.M. Stronge, P. Klima,
B. Horner

ACKNOWLEDGEMENTS

Some of these poems have appeared in
Descant, Malahat Review, Canadian Literature, The Australian,
and *The Tasmanian Literary Reporter*

Cobalt 3 is named for the
Radiation Room in the Cancer Control Agency
in Vancouver where Kevin Roberts
was treated for non-Hodgkin's Lymphoma.

CONTENTS

After John Donne

Every man is an island
and each woman too

single and slippery
as conception, grains
as separate as thumbprints
or the unique voice
print here on the page

Oh, don't bother to tell me
I'm richer not alone
for all the birds of a feather
solidarity is not sung in one voice

and though the eroding sea
has its wicked way with promontories
washing them slice by slice into its will
which diminisheth not

a single dove flew the flood
to a single island of peace

and every song cries against the grain
tossed in the crevice of time

for the sea flushes us to islands
the absolute and bloody best way
it can.

Naturally

Naturally you don't believe it

the first lump, ah, just a bug sting
bad beer, the other couple of buds
too much Aussie shiraz wine
or an allergy

you take an antihistamine
and naturally, forget it

but they grow like tiny
barnacles under your skin
on your neck, in your groin

naturally you don't take them seriously
you reckon they'll subside

but like damn little oyster seeds
they start stringing together

so you drop in to the Clinic, ask
for penicillin, reckon that'll fix
anything unnatural
you've ever had before

but the doc's got a frown
as he fingers the little lumps
tells you you'd better
get one cut out for a look see

naturally you figure he's a nervous Nelly
and these little mushrooms'll
die off like weeds in winter
but naturally they don't
he's right

naturally you get this flutter
a hummingbird trapped in your chest
flying the length
of a high white wall
unnaturally brick by solid
brick right in front
of your nose

Biopsy

you never make the countdown
or hear the end of the surgeon's story
Englishman, Scot, German
as the anaesthetist counts 10, 9, you
buzz out at 5 or 4, drop
into some deep black sack

wake up sick with a maniac
twist of knife in your neck

you don't remember the drive home
wake up in bed in a fuzz of light
your doc's there, your wife, eyes huge
behind him, he sits on the bed
tells you the biopsy result
you just dumb nod, numb as your bedstead

Later it seeps in, this whisper, you've
got cancer, this chant, cancer
you've got cancer, thunders
in your head, but all you can remember

is that one teal in the flight of dozens
off the lagoon in Barmera, you're fourteen
your first shotgun
one quick unaimed blast
and that one unlucky duck slip-slides

frantic, picked by some unknown finger
to drop, flailing out of the sky.

Journey

One day the sun simply
drops

behind my feet the dark cliff crumbles
but I scramble up higher
grab a quick look
at a land I have never believed in
before

one shaving of light
far, far away, flickers
bright yellow
in the monstrous dark

about me
a forest of writhing trees
aphoristic flowers
unspeakable weeds

in front loom mountains
sharp peaks   deep black valleys
rivers of turbulent ebony

beyond a dark snake sea
writhes
under one fragile butterfly
of red gold luminescence
fading as I watch

time is the essence
and in this land there are no
maps

but somewhere I know there is a path
a direction
I must find on my own

I take a deep breath
fix my sight on the yellow light

take the first urgent step

Narrows

We walk by the Narrows
follow some leader or habit or fad
single file on a narrow path by a cliff edge, below
the flood tide, 9 knots, whirlpools away
into the dusk

but someone or thing, maybe
you yourself, kicks your heels
you drop
flail in the rapids

you yell for help, go under, yell
again, but no one up there
has a rope or life ring
though rows of them stare,
a few wave, a bunch crouch
for a better view, one or two cry out
as you swirl away.

At first you're frantic
swim madly for the shore
but you're too weak
in the tide rip's
all mindless muscle
you tread water
suck down into a whirlpool
pop up, gasp, spot a man in a white coat
on a nearby rock holding out a red lifejacket
you grab, whizz by, a bit steadier
but the scrum of tide topples you

you glance desperately downstream
see another white figure
knee deep in a back eddy

he swings out a lasso and you know
you've got one chance to grab it

your hand burns into the rope
but he can't haul you in

and you swing
in the wild water, learn to hang there
for the many hours the tide takes
to run its course.

Phone Calls

The first few times the phone rings
you blow it

No one knows what to say
and you're no help
too angry, scared and bitter
to bother with sentiment, besides
they all seem to have written you
off.

Finally you sense they've all
written it down like a script.
they're reading it to you
over the phone, prepared
edited and rehearsed for days

and you realize they're more scared than you
because you at least have felt
the beast grow its serrated tail
within you, but like a leper
you've nearly touched them
with unimagined sores
and their rosy lens has just
dropped a couple of future
f-stops

and suddenly you feel
sorry for them, for their flesh
and their fumbling
attempts at concern

you get a bit stronger
if not wiser, and then the one
call from Australia, so brash
it's real, *"Hey, Blue, what's this*
I hear about you and the big C?
I'm bloody glad it's you and not me
old mate!"

And you relax and laugh
at last, at the stupid honest horror
of it all.

Role

They've watched too much of it
TV screen bulges smoke and clouds
angels in double-breasted suits, Oxford accents
fateful roles in bright afterdeath
all caring fathers hover over kids
quarterbacks in altered states toss
the Hail Mary pass in a ghostly Super Bowl

It's like a bad TV role, as soon
as the word gets out, you're playing
everybody's script, books turn up
gifts from anxious friends
"how to" "hands on" life
books with ironic titles
like "Death the Final Growth"
advising you how to
tuck Dad into the casket yourself, dig
his grave, shovel the dirt in personally

Stanislavsky method, get involved
and feel better, accept your part in the play
Death carves out on stone with a blunt
chisel

Damn it, it's bad enough some unknown judge
advised a bored jury
threw a black cap on his head
tossed you behind bars, waiting
for the final drop, while your friends
drown you in sympathy or avert their eyes

you want your old role with them
back, but they expect
butterfly grace and the best you can do
is imitate a crawling chemo caterpillar

And you realize, suddenly, you're a professional
actor in a role
unrehearsed
that everybody
plays only once.

Marrow

Like an oil spill the seep
of crooked cells runs iridescent
romps in the streams of blood
corrupts the soft lymph glands set
to fight the cancer's gag and throttle grip
but it oozes, finally into the marrow

Today you wait on your side
on a white clinic bed
for the marrow test

The doc's done this 1,000 times, chats
as he flips up your green coat
you grip the thin rails in the bedstead

a quick prick, the flesh on your hip
freezes distant and dumb

strangely foreign and far off
the big needle bites into mute
flesh, then, a sudden punch
chunk that shudders your whole
frame, steel stuck in your very
bone

your fists grip the bedstead
needle digs ice cold hole in your hip

doc pulls the plunger up, still
chatty, your teeth grind down
he retracts, you flop like a gunshot
deer
he walks off with a pink
snowstorm of marrow in the tube.

You lie quivering.
The nurse
arrives to clean you up, says
*"Good Lord, you've bent
the bedstead."*

Insurance

Great West Insurance man
sweet olive oil on the phone
Freedom 55, you and your lady
on Waikiki forever, he offers
paw paw and pineapple bliss, says
you really must update for your estate
you're not getting any younger
you almost hear the palm trees
wave, see white sand and surf break
over the phone

you sense instead
the Damoclean sword hover, begin
to spin
over your head

You give him a minute more

He pauses, sure of closing, you
tell him flatly, you've got cancer
wait through the silence
he mumbles, hangs up

you have a minute of self-disgust
like an ice hockey cheap shot
you blind-sided the guy
put his head into the boards
you give yourself a game misconduct

you're not proud of cruelty

but damn it, he had
your future sold for silver
anyway.

Conference

you sit like a prisoner
green uniform, in a cubicle

one by one, the docs come in
check you against the file
British pleasantries, old chap
occasionally a quick feel
and they're off to meet
determine your treatment, your fate

You wait.
Imagine the long table of docs
figuring statistics, medic history
probability, dicing your chances
against the pills, poison, cobalt light

Finally your doc comes in, your guru
he's a bit downcast, tells you
they won't go for the radical stuff

you want to jump up and burst
through their closed door, thump
the table, demand the toughest
shot they've got

but all this techno probability, stats, recovery rates
sounds like modern witchcraft
has you bluffed, bamboozled
so instead you nod, he leaves

you dress, leave the Cancer Clinic

walk down 7th for a block or two
peering blindly in the window
of the Future Shop
pretending you're just another
shopper, hunting for bargains
on some surrealistic sidewalk.

Chemotherapy — Lion's Gate

Two of us today in the Chemo Room
drip fed, pampered like premie babies
in our high chairs
the plastic tubes needled
into our veins, the bags
of chemicals hung in chrome stands
high above our heads, glug slowly
down from over our heads

Today I'm hooked to a green bag, he's
on red, Jimmy Jones' Kool Aid
Kids we joke, my hair
thinning more than his dark
thick mop

And an auxiliary lady
sparse grey hair under a net
wanders in, wheeling a tray
offering cookies and magazines and pop
smiles, says cheerfully, to him

*"My, your hair
is lasting well"*

And with a bitter grin
he yanks out a thick handful
hands it to the stunned woman
says

*"Here, you need it
more than me."*

Betrayal

No matter what the books tell you
or the full care voices of lovers

You're on your own.

cut out from the herd
dropped from the songs and ceremonies
spun off while the green blue
planet turns graciously away

cuckolded by your own flesh

like living with someone
you never suspected before
was secretly a whore
you lie awake at 3 a.m.
with this slut of a body
snoring its gangly bones
of deceit within you

you can't even see
the raucous party in your own
bawdy blood, as the cells gang bang away
dumb glands grinning as they spread
wide, and have it on behind the host's
back, abandoned to the animal moment
while your future and theirs flops
on the screen into a fade, lap and dissolve.

you know the only way out
is family violence
you have to
damn near kill yourself
to clean up their act
open up to radiation
to vomit and shit them out
or poison the mad beast with chemo
in selfish revenge
like some bad Elizabethan play

just to get back respect, yes
just that chance to start again

breathe in the blue bright air
all those about you
walk and talk in without thinking
take so easily
for granted.

Prudent

The Prudent Disability Company
is naturally sceptical
doesn't really believe
you're sick
reckons you're faking it
secretly partying and laughing
behind their responsible backs

and they're trying to catch you out
trap you in a slip or a lie or a grey shade
of sly truth, so they can cut
you off their beneficent list

and somewhere behind the slim
envelopes and embossed letterhead
questions that arrive every month
is a face, hands that type
the same cold interrogations

When were you first diagnosed?
Who are your doctors?
When did you cease work?
When will you return to work?
What are your other sources of income?

all answers they've had ten times before
but every month the same squares/ticks/dates
to fill out, the same imponderables
that really ask when will you die
and satisfy our statistical bottom line?

questions you dare not mess with
because they love delay
and double check return verification
before the cheque reluctantly arrives

and you want to turn up at
Prudent's Head Office, glide
up to the fifth floor, strip
naked and stand on the desk
of the face and hands
that question your pain
force them to touch

like doubting Thomas
the tiny globules of dissent

thrust their hands on to your
radiation burns

while you shake your falling hair

all over their doubting neat desk.

Conman

He sidles up to you
clipped white moustache
Harris tweed and tie

"Alternatives," he whispers, *"chemicals and radiation
don't always work. Now almonds"*
he says, *"essence of almonds
in Mexico. Or natural chemicals
the magic spa waters of Belgium
to correct the body's mistakes."*

You sit there in your ironic green
gown, while under you an imagined iron grating
is greased and sliding ever so slowly
and silently open. You want badly
to believe that out there someone
holds the cure in a gold cup of grace
you can kneel before and worship

because you can't afford to think
this is a slippery
dip you're on.
You take his card.
think how it can't hurt to enquire.

But you know there are no Belgian angels
hovering passionately overhead
to fly you back into light
or magic Mexican brews to zap
you back to health
and Darwin logged the tree
of eternal life 100 years ago.

No. It's up to you
and you tear the card into tiny pieces
toss it in the trash can when you walk
wide eyed into room
Cobalt No. 3

Shooting Up

She slaps your wrist, finds the right
vein
a quick sliver of pain, needle
like a dart quivers
on top of your clenched hand

the first shot is for nausea
clear, cold as vodka, a shooter
squeezed in through the dart
taped tight to the top
of your hand, you feel it
run about your body, tingle
in your jaw

And your dealer walks in, white coat
tapping a green, blue or red bag
of tricks, chemo, hair dust-off
joint ache, mind scatter of rainbow
poison, kills the good the bad
and the ugly with indifference

But you're connected
taped in, screwed down
to the last drip
of gravity
red bag above, your flag
hung on a steel stand
white wheels at its base

you can sit or walk but the bag
hangs on like Sinbad's sailor

And you don't dare break this habit
you're hooked, dumb as a dogfish
grateful as a Lab
to this plastic bag and tube

Ariadne's ball of twine
leading all the way back to light.

Chipmunk

"Look, Mum," little kid in Safeway
all grave sincerity, points at me,
"He looks like Charley Chipmunk"

the mother's hush and blush, she
glances up from the kid

But you've got to laugh
8 pills a day
2 bags of green poison a week
a chemo bloat
of a body, a cheek bulge big
as Satchmo on his trumpet

you look like a grotesque refugee from
a Breughel peasant painting

But if only you could find
the golden nuts the Gods
have squirrelled away

crack the shell and eat
the magic acorn of health

Tricks with Lights

He talks you into meditation
the mind he says
can make you sick
but also cure you

lie back he says
he loosens his holy collar
says imagine a bright
white bar of love
whispers, focus the light
lower it down your head, neck
chest, belly, push
the bad cells down to where
you can flush them out

You try that for a day or two
but you're too angry, aggressive
get mad at its sad, gentle Jesus
meek and mild light
invent your own great
white sharks, imagine them
luminous in your blood and flesh
whipping frenziedly about
chopping up, tearing
gulping down the fucked-up cells
imagine the sharks, full guts
churning from your head to your toes
zooming out your urine stream

your own deadly
slim white sharks
of hope

Ferry Ride

Two dolphins at play in the spray
ride the carve of the wave at the bow
of the *Queen of Nanaimo*

how their slick shapes shimmer
in and out of the green bend
of sea
And I am jealous that they know
how to twist force
to their will, bodies easy with power
they roll and turn in the wave

I am travelling to kill cells
strap myself in for a dose
of chemicals glugged into my veins
pumped through my blood

caught in
this wave of destruction
I must ride the curve of pain
surf in the white crest
away from the steel bow

like these dolphins easy
in their flesh
ride the way back
to the calm waters
of Departure Bay

Cinéma-Vérité

It's like bad boys and cops on TV
a raid and arrests

I assume the position
in this badly written script
hands up, legs spread

pat me down, oh sage
detect my lumpy cells
empty my pockets of flesh
strip search my blood

play that good cop bad cop
red and green chemical rag
again and again

cuff me in my green
hospital coat of many colours
I will sell out and betray
for any shortened
sentence, perjure, bear false witness
live a.k.a., anonymous anywhere

but I gather this
is the final appeal
and no Governor will make a last
minute call
while I sit in my chair

turn up the gas
fire up the atoms, blow
light from above

o radiance o dome
of single-hued misery

let poison and fire
celebrate my desire

then round up the usual suspects.

Terra Incognita

On its nightly rounds the black ship drops me off.
I row to my island, unroll my medicine bundle, check supplies

I sleep in my inherited cabin, at dawn inspect the walls
scrawled with ciphers, initials, questions in strange tongues

Outside my porch, a galaxy of islets spin
to the horizon, too far to swim, every way I turn
tiny figures gesticulate like puppets on far shores

Each rock, my daily bread, I drop
one after the other over the edge
and so my breakwater grows, stone
by slow stone, to the next isle
Will my island hold rocks enough to fill the deep?

By night, I float my green messages out in flasks
By day, unfold absurd notes bottled by unknown hands

Only one writes the rumour of the great white ship
To sail one dawn to free us, no note says why or when.

Shield

She fits you for your shield
tape measure about her neck
mouth pursed like a seamstress
she checks your nakedness
bare to the bone
against an x-ray of kidneys
lungs heart

no bronze dragons, pennants, embossed lions rampant
this shield is lead
curves and squares to fit up into
the cobalt light

and her bright Brit voice again
"Do you have a family coat of arms?"
the cold tape end touches my heart
"No," I say, *"only family jewels
and will you protect them?"*
but she only giggles, says
she's giving me a brand new
shield, one off, uniquely mine

"And now for the hero part," she smiles
*"something special to remember me
forever,"* and she produces a needle
black ink, pricks two tattoos
one low in the groin, one high
on the chest, *"To line you up"*
she says, *"in the spotlight for the fray."*

Last thing on your mind, the glory
of battle, forget the Greeks and Achilles
brought back splendid on his shield

You're in a back alley fight
with only teeth and nails and boots
and all you want to do
is crawl out of it
alive.

Alternatives

It seems to make them happy
their oddball cures and their conviction
and you don't know what to say
or do with their concern
these awkward visitors perched
earnestly on your chesterfield

though you know they see their own faces
in your frightened eyes

but you're ready to flip any card
toss any dice

and a little stream of caregivers
like anxious ants
or lost magi
turn up at your door
bearing gifts

the first one's organic
carries bottles of carrot
and spinach juice
the iron and carotin to flush
all the bad shit from your blood

the second one's an advocate of the sea
from which, at one time
she says we all arose

pushes bottles of pills
white and red, into your hands
kelp and seaweed and pure sea
salt to scatter the cancer from my flesh

the third one's cautious, slow to mention
that at the local Anglican Church
your friends, mindful of your
considerably lapsed Christian morals
include you in their weekly prayer group
and you're grateful if bemused
and thankful, mainly, they don't expect
you to join in

the fourth one slips a baggy
of marijuana into your top pocket
"The best stuff," he says, *"just the tips*
to relax your mind, man
chill out, let it all go, straighten up"
he sucks back a big gust
of Gabriola Gold
winks, says, *"toke up, my man*
toke up and get well."

Ski-Slope Doc

"Sure, they'll find the golden bullet,"
says a young doc, intern, fresh cheeked
from a Whistler weekend
"it's only a matter of time."

He checks your chart, tells you about
his time, damn near Olympic, full bore
downhill, checks you with confident hands

you remember that confidence in flesh
once, watch him rush away

leaving you
with only time, so much time in
some blind hourglass, flipped by casual fingers
so much time on your hands, in your
blood, time and no space for Odyssean
quests, time ticking on a chart
a computer, a Sisyphean hill
and you going downhill as slow as hell
with every brake you have
stuck on hard
and smoking to beat hell.

Monster

Blue jeans three sizes too big
hung with fireman's braces
to put out the fire of
irritated skin burnt from chemo
radiation, an Extra OS shirt to keep
any rub of arms, shoulders, back
at bay

your face bloats up
to suit this new inside image
balding redneck, hippy hick
off a Hornby Island farm
Cat hat jammed tight to hide
the falling hair

but the worst is the knot
of poisoned
protein in your fingernails
that flattens the tips
then curls them up at the edges
so they shatter at the scissor's edge
like glass
grow concave, writhe
at your fingertips

and your toenails spread
crooked as arbutus trunks
brittle as sugar, twist and shout
against your shoes

all this ugly ducking
from the mirror
looking through the glass
at the green grass field
of health.

Cobalt 3

They shuffle him in
shackles clinking
green gown and handcuffs
past the queue of patients
two prison guards, nightsticks
dangling, for even criminals must be burnt
well
and you watch the guards stare
through thick glass at him
shackled and prone
under the sacrificial light

and you, in your bottle green
hospital gown, green slippers and cap
next

the bald and halt and just damned sick
wait their turn for the sacred glowworm
crouched against a huge mural of crocuses
daffodils, in a green field
somewhere in a country smelling
of health.

Ashen-faced, he's helped out
the lead doors,
you willingly
walk in past the nuke sign
lie down, as the squares of light
line up on your tattoos, one
on your chest, one
on your groin, pulled and pushed
you stay still, the young nurses

joke and hustle out the lead
door

All there is now, the freezing overhead buzz
later, vomit and shit
but the nurse says,
"This is mirror art" as she draws
a red dahlia on your bum
giggles, and all you can do
is laugh, but later, the toilet
stuck tight to your shaking
body, you think you might have to
demand handcuffs and shackles, too,
next time.

Ferry

17 shots of full frontal
radiation, your blood count
dicier than any penny stock
on the the Vancouver Stock Exchange
they send you home to eat spinach
like Popeye

your wife's eyes
try to betray nothing, ignore
your skinned rabbit frame
head hair thinning
body skin hairless
as a baby, and about as steady
on your pins

And on the *Queen of Nanaimo*
you get up to go for two coffees

fall flat on your face, hear
the whispers, *"Drunk before Noon"*
"Disgraceful"
your wife tries

to help you up, you push
her away, angry at this damn
creak and groan of flesh
you've come to

Almost wish for the Captain
to march down from the bridge
shove the coin on your tongue
cut you loose in a lifeboat
out into easy
darkness.

Interns

Three of them are waiting when I turn up.
The nurse slaps a green gown in my hand.
"I would prefer white," I say, she sniggers
says, *"Green suits your florid complexion."*
"Not to mention," you add, *"my fading red hair?"*
(what's left of it, sweetie, she thinks)

"Just get undressed," she says, flat as a used
spatula, whisks the green curtain across

and I enter my island of floating flesh
lie down like a lamb in open green
as the line of interns forms outside

three at a time, not a gang grope this, but
serious medical experience, a hands-on
fingering of non-Hodgkin's fickle rosary of lumps.

The first one can't find anything.
An Asian girl, Coke-bottle glasses
her Mum's told her not to touch
anywhere near there, she jerks
away at first, then I
guide her tiny hand, clear nails, slim fingers
trembling to the string of pearl
lumps in my neck, my belly, my groin
her hand like a wren fluttering in fear
near my cock, *"C'mon,"* I say, *"It won't bite
but you've got to feel under,"* and her
tiny fingers flash in for a furtive
second, and *"No,"* I say, *"not those two
the tiny ones underneath,"* and she
pulls back, puts her hands behind her back.

The next one's a big hairy jock
tries to push in against my hand
can't feel a thing, and *"Listen, mate"*
I say, *"It's like making love, the softer*
the touch, the more you'll get in return"
and his paws relax a bit, finally get on
to the puffed up vanity row of cells.

But the third one, a girl with cinnamon eyes
cool hands, has it, instantly, glances at my face
the moment her forefinger touches the first
grape globe, and I nod, and she senses also
the freeway pileup, chain collision, knows the slow
crash of dumb cells, sees in my eyes how
they screech and smash, feels
the brawl in my blood hears
the silent screams in my head.

Disappearing Trick

I am disappearing for you
in your script of this film

watch out for me
I could jump out
jack-in-a-box you 3-D dead
centre

But I am disappearing for you
into the light   it's easy
this trick, Hey Presto, natural
as day, this dissolve into
white light, the white thighs
the white face, white
cells

I am self-effacing in this next
cut, drip by red bag drip
vanishing hair, protruding ribs

I am disappearing from you
my tan knees, my dark feet
worm into the solemn
earth

But it's too easy, when the cloak
flies wide, and the white
bones slide apart
quicker than lime

so let us cross fade
to another scene

where you
are disappearing from me
into a swirl of fog

and the film burns a white
hole on the screen
the projector runs wild
in an endless flop
and clatter of broken film.

Survivor

His hands are leather pouches
over steel, draught horse shoulders
famous Cat hat strength
he can heave the 17-ft Campion straight
on its trailer, hold in one hand
a 24-inch Husquavarna bucking up maple
in a scurr of wood chips

He gets it the same time as you

You figure he'll do it easy time

But when you talk, his eyes drift
off, it's the chemicals he says,
no damn good, a man feels
weak all the time, can't lift or push
or carry or pull, can't fish or hunt
or cut the winter firewood.

You decide to swim with it, he
fights every inch
thrashes upstream
while you retreat
into a stubborn redoubt, he attacks
the unseen

Both of you losing hair, muscles
shrinking back to bone, toe nails
twist grotesque.

He shakes his head
struggles harder   goes under you
dies in eight months.
you curse in fear
grab harder on the rope
dangling over the pit
afraid you'll be tempted like him
to take the tough shit
easy drop
into the dark

No Plath Please

When I climbed back, they unstrung a banner
"Welcome back," they echoed and cheered
crowded in to pinch my arms and tug my new hair.
"Wow, it's really you," they shrieked and slapped

each other on the back, hi-fived and jigged
for the victory was theirs more than mine
and knowing this I carried my mirrored shield
slung to the ground I'd escaped, so no one's face

appeared, but their celebration was short lived — edgy
one by one they got me aside, cried, *"Well? Tell us!
What did you see? How close did you get? How come
you've got no scars? Was the face as we imagined?"*

Shook their heads at my explanations, gathered again
in disbelief, till I held the mirror shield high, but all they saw
was the reflection of Medusa's freezing stare.

The Maze

One morning you wake up
inside this maze

endless narrow
paths
thorn bushes stretch out
mesmeric   manicured
twice your height
blind turns and right
angles
under a weak sun fumbling
across the sky

no exit   no entrance
and no fix on the eight
spun compass points
to guide your silent path
and only torn rags on the sharp thorns
tells you others have stumbled this way

no idea how to escape
and you can only keep
walking straight ahead, keep
your head up, keep walking, guess
left or right, keep walking
scared to turn back
or admit you're lost

you keep turning   guess
right or left
walk right up to the thick
thorns
turn one way
keep walking.

Photo

My moth of memory flutters, lost
in the bright past, swims up
one precious photo
polaroid, black and white

My brother Malcolm, slim
cotton-shirted traveller, smiling
back from Holy Toledo and Spain
woollen shoulder bag, fisherman's cap
arm around a girl
in Sloane Square, London, 1972

a week before he flew
back to Adelaide, back
to a terminal marriage
before the girl swallowed sleeping pills
in his Torrens flat
before he showed the lumps
to his doctor, and a week later took
the deep breath in the white winged hospital
into the black sleep and scalpel

and a week later, John
my eldest brother, phones me in Devon
tells me he's sitting
next to a vase of white roses
by the white hospital bed

next to Malcolm, who lifts his green gown
shows blood black scars all over his white
skinny frame, cries

"They cut me," John
surprised as a little boy
he says, *"they cut me all over
here and here,"* he traces
the dark stitches, and John
unable to speak

a week before Malcolm crumbles
into speechless dust

and 5,000 miles away
in an English spring
I sit in my student carrel
in Exeter, curse and cry
because I'm too broke
to fly back to Adelaide

cutjump the film
to 15 years later, and I'm lying
in a green gown under a white
hot flower in Vancouver
Malcolm's image grey in my eyes
before the black cobalt moth buzzes
white in its lead cage

hoping the light burns
the moth of fear in my gut
before my brother's lumps
reach through my genes to betray
my soft winged breath to dust

hoping the flash camera
burns away the negative

slides out a clear photo
in full Kodak colour

Statistics

1.

Crude Stats   Per 100,000

Time magazine announces cancer cure success

1990   135 per 100,000
1996   130 per 100,000
Breast cancer down 6.2%
Prostate cancer down 6.2%

cheery figures
but sex levels the field

uterus 20%   prostate 20%
a bitter equality   bizarre
finger flipped up at our genesis

But who knows these other people
dead certs, the poor sods
workers like the women in the 1920 factory

who earned their deadly daily bread
by dipping their brushes in radium paint
and diligently licking the tips
to a fine point
to paint the hours of the day
twelve at a time
on the luminous dials of watches

and the truth of statistics denies each
bone-tight suffering face
the frail fingers curled on skinny laps
machinists and millwrights and carpenters
and miners and secretaries and engineers

a deadly democracy in chemical and paint factories
asbestos and copper mines, refineries and farms
or just on Vancouver streets

all breathing in Thanatos

like the obedient soldiers who squatted
to attention in their Los Alamos slit trenches
in 1945, to observe, unprotected
the first atomic blast
and its winged rush of death
over their bowed heads

Stats 2.

She gets it in the soft
bulges of her breasts
small milk curve of flesh
low blow at female vanity

she plays tennis like a ballet dancer
feet light as air

she phones to cancel the doubles
tells me she's just got her test back
and it's so bad she says she's not going to bother
with chemo or radiation
because it'll just make her last months
on earth painful and miserable
and she cannot stand the thought
of losing her breast, the indignity
the ugly bones breaking through
the bald skull, the white shell of skin
fleshless arms   she's seen it
hates it   the feral regression

I rage back at her, talk quickly
yes, angrily yes, madly yes, you can

she's surprised at my voice
falters and agrees
goes through the black
waterfall   yelling and kicking
hidden in scarves and sunglasses

and a year later she pirouettes
on the tennis court
her dark hair fans wide, she
slams a forehand
down the tramlines, leaves me
standing stuck at the net

she dances back to serve
giggling
and alive

Stats 3.

He gets it in the head
mushroom bullet blooming
right on that diamond spot
where his famed wit
glances glittering through
all the facets of his quick brain, explodes
into rainbow laughter

He's always been ahead of the game
elder statesman, *consigliore*
guardian of his mates

but it hits him at home
slices his syntax slurs the bright words
his speech turn of phrase   won't
come   easily   hardly
at all
and his arms and legs go
slow motion

I phone him to coach, cajole, bullshit him
back, but his battery's low on juice, I hear
on the phone his words slow as snail trails
his will crinkling like an old birthday balloon

I can only imagine the brilliant cracks
in his flashing opal mind   hear it fade
like a single frame caught in a sprocket
flowering burnt celluloid
to white

The Flesh

At 5:35 a.m. the sun splits the dark
wide open   spits
red light between the firs
blues the seething sea

You haven't slept
thinking of the white light
the endless fight
waiting for you across the heaving swell

four more radiation shots
and maybe you've beaten it off
enough to join the energy of all the flesh
teeming about you

out in Nanoose Bay
the salmon's silver dash
into the speckled herring flash
explodes the school   bits
of herring float up
in a shiny star burst

for the seagulls to plummet
into the boil of white water and flesh

and open mouthed, the ling cod
mouth gapes wide open for spinning
fragments

and crows patrol the shore
pick open the soft sores of shells

and above them like crucifixions
eagles hang
in the white turning air
drop down for whatever flesh
flounders in the tideline

all this furious fight for food, survival
you know you're part of, but you
can't eat, knowing the cobalt light
will churn your stomach into a wash
cycle slosh in just a few hours

you sip coffee, watch through the window
humming birds
at the blood red feeder
young musketeers crossing
their beaks like swords
in this shrill and frantic fight

to reach beyond our solitary flesh

Ten Green Bottles

The nurses clip by quick and clean
starched white uniforms
order in their trim shapes
practised smiles

They all march with such confident
strides, their roles
important and sharp
as their triangular hats

You sit with a sprawl
of nine other patients
in a row of seats
against a white wall
waiting in green hospital gowns
your slippers unsure, slipping
on the polished linoleum floor

The docs saunter by in twos and threes
white housecoats flaring, ties, jackets
you catch a snippet of a golf game
or the Vegas vacation, or the new BMW

You admire the square of their lives
the cut tight system they control
their ship shape mathematical pattern
in this maelstrom of disease

the belief so sure in the future
you hear one doc say he's enrolled
his newborn already
in some private British school

you try to understand
how they live by measuring disorder
balancing probabilities of flesh
drip feeding decay
yet seem untouched

you try to bridge the gap
between their flesh and yours
imagine the minute cancer cells
raving in their flesh

they seem impervious
untouchable, as solid as the concrete
wall at your back

but you know
you're just one of the ten
green bottles on the wall
and you hope it's not you
who'll accidentally fall.

Check Up

The waiting gets to you

You begin to hate the ferry ride
1 hr 45 minute hollow drum
the *Queen of Somewhere* vibrating
30 miles across the Straight

Below the sea moves
in endless whitecaps
mountains razorback, immutable
blue sky, you can only imagine
losing all this
but all you can grasp
is six months' magic remission

furtively, you check your neck
armpits, groin for tiny lumps

two hours later you're naked
under a green gown, waiting,
not reading *Maclean's.*

The doc's in fast, quick fingers
trace of a grin, karate push
into your stomach and off

you dress, wait in his office
listen to the phone as he
grave faced, kisses off
someone else, turns to you.
You ask him the big question. He
can't answer it. You leave.

But Hell, you're alive
a reprieve for another six months
You forget the elevator, skip
down all the stairs, jump
the building's steps
like Rocky, spin, raise
your hands to the wild sun.

Decrapitation

the hot light fades
on clear plastic memory
yellows and cracks
breaks in the sun, blows
into fog   swims in lazy and thick

the curtain falls, the director shouts
cut, that's a wrap
and all the frames coil up
tight in a can, shoved away
on some dusty shelf

you forget

the rat stink fear, muscletight
chest, watery flush in your belly
hair fallen on your pillow
hairless groin, puffed up baby face
the coppery panic taste

you carry your bag of tricks back to work
turn the key in your office door
sit at your desk, as if nothing happened

but outside the landscape has mutated
the sure dark path down   tilts upward
to a weird sunlit hill ahead

and you don't dare look back
for fear that all you've won
will turn to pillars of salt in the fog

But you can still fast rewind
appointments, dates, hospitals
doctors, nurses, attendants, friends
in the film noir you starred in
but never want to see again

and you're surprised
the dromedary world has gone on
in its dull trot of timetables, meetings, deadlines
the impossible marathon in and out
of the endless mundane maze

but the shadow rat sleeps still
in your flesh, wakes some nights
scurries in the tunnels of your bones
and you jolt bolt upright
into a role you know
you never want to play again

Lunch

The first time back at work
you don't want to go to lunch
but someone talks you into it
says they'll all be pleased to see you

but you're not sure
feel their glances
like needles

eyes measuring your flesh
whispers tallying
your mortal coil, you smell
their dismay, know some are confused
by your return, had you
neatly buried, written and crossed
off their books and you've thrown
their certain bets back into the bookie's bag

you sense the question
unheard   hovering

of your weird survivor guilt
why you should have made it
and others not

and they think you carry death
like an overdue Mastercard
in your hip pocket

while others avoid your eyes
mix their fear with yours

of this capricious snake
invisible to human eyes
coiling up to rainbow
its subtle but careless fangs
into anyone passing by.

ABOUT THE AUTHOR

Kevin Roberts came to Canada from Adelaide, South Australia in 1966. After completing his Masters Degree in English at Simon Fraser University he began teaching at Malaspina University College when it opened in 1969. He has studied in England and lived in Greece. For five years he ran a 32-foot salmon troller in Georgia Straight and on the West Coast. In 1985 he was Writer in Residence at Wattle Park College in Adelaide, and trekked into the outback of the Northern Territory. In 1997 he was a Visiting Professor in English at Rajamangala Institute of Technology at Nan in Northern Thailand.

From 1987 to 1991 he went through two chemotherapy treatments for non-Hodgkin's Lymphoma. When these failed, he was given 21 shots of radiation treatment, which was successful in obtaining remission. He now lives with his wife Maria and sons Anthony and Jonathan on Sunset Beach, on Vancouver Island, and teaches English and Creative Writing at Malaspina University College.